# Best Varicose Vein Treatments

"Discover Little Know Natural Remedies For Varicose Veins"

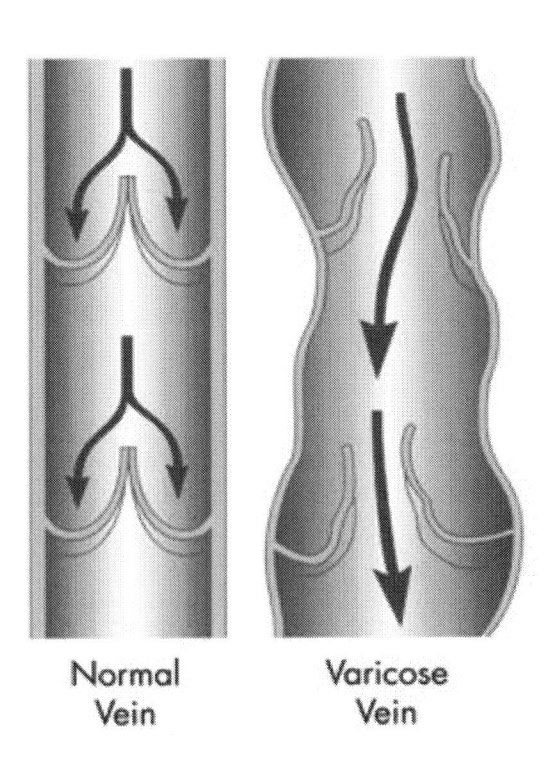

Normal Vein

Varicose Vein

Rudy S Silva, Natural Nutritionist

Best Varicose Vein Treatments? © 2012 by Rudy S Silva

ISBN-13: 978-1481955836

ISBN-10: 1481955837

Disclaimer and Terms of Use: All Rights Reserved. No part of this publication may be reproduced in any form or by any means, including scanning, photocopying, or otherwise without prior written permission of the copyright holder.

The Author and Publisher has strived to be as accurate and complete as possible in the creation of this book, notwithstanding the fact that he does not warrant or represent at any time that the contents within are accurate due to the rapidly changing nature of the Internet. While all attempts have been made to verify information provided in this publication, the Author and Publisher assumes no responsibility for errors, omissions, or contrary interpretation of the subject matter herein. Any perceived slights of specific persons, peoples, or organizations are unintentional. In practical advice books, like anything else in life, there are no guarantees of income made.

All readers are advised to seek their own medical help.

The information here is for educational purposes and in no way is it medical advice or treatment. Ask your doctor before using any of the natural remedies listed here.

First Printing, 2012 Printed in the United States of America

# Table of Contents

1: What Are Varicose Veins All About? 5

2: Do You Know What Causes Varicose Veins? 9

3: What Foods Will Fight Your Varicose Veins? 15

4: Constipation Remedies That Stop Varicose Veins 19

5: How Varicose Veins Are Created By An Acid Body 27

6: Most Powerful Supplements for Varicose Veins 33

7: Effective Natural Remedies For Varicose Veins 37

8: Final Comments On Varicose Veins 45

9: Resources You Need To Know About 49

# 1: What Are Varicose Veins All About?

There are around 80 million Americans that have varicose veins. They occur more frequently in women over the age of 50. If your parents suffered from them, then chances you will too, and they may occur when you are much younger.

The formation of varicose veins does not occur all of a sudden, when you turn 50. It's a process that is slowly progressing from an early age. That is why this is a preventable condition, just like so many other body conditions or illnesses.

The word varicose comes from Latin varix, which means twisted. If you have varicose veins, you see that they are twist and spread across your legs. They can appear thin or large and can cover a small or large area. Varicose veins occur when the valve in your veins, nears the surface of your skin, stop working.

**Valves In Your Veins**

These valves are designed to move blood from your legs to your heart, using your leg muscles. As your leg muscles contract, the vein valves open and blood is sent up your veins toward your heart. The valves then close preventing blood from flowing back down toward your feet.

If the valves malfunction and do not close, blood will move back into your veins and collect causing the veins to stretch. Eventually a bulging of the veins occurs and these bluish or gray veins become visible through the skin.

Varicose veins are uncomfortable and painful. They ache and swell and will get worse over time. Varicose vein can occur anywhere in your body, when they occur around your anus, they are called hemorrhoids.

## Removing Varicose Veins

Aside from being painful, varicose veins are not attractive. If you find it difficult to reduce their appearance or to get rid of them, using natural remedies, then the only alternative is to have surgical treatment. Laser application is also possible.

The small spider veins can be removed with laser therapy or by injection therapy of sclerotherapy. Here the doctor injects fatty acids with salt water into the affected area, which causes the veins to collapse.

For the larger varicose veins a surgical procedure called mini-phlebotomy or stripping can be used. In this procedure, the surgeon makes a cut and inserts a wire hook and pulls out the veins. It will take you a few weeks to recover from this procedure.

Despite the surgery, varicose veins tend to come back, if you have not taken the steps to eliminate the causes. In this e-book you will find the many causes for varicose and what you need to do to eliminate these causes.

There is no known drug therapy for correcting and healing various veins. But there are many natural remedies that can help to minimize the size of these veins and even get rid of them, if they are not severe. It will require patience and trial and error in what remedies you try. The healing time will not be fast and will take up to 3 months or longer to see some results. But it will be worth using a natural remedy and nutrition process, which can result in a side effect of better health.

## Thrombophlebitis

Varicose veins are not a condition to ignore, since they can lead to more serious conditions. From varicose veins, a condition can develop call phlebitis, where veins become painfully inflamed. If you ignore this condition, it can develop into thrombophlebitis, where blood clots form in the affected area.

If a small clot breaks off, it will travel to your lungs and pose a threat to your life. If you encounter, painful swelling in your legs that doesn't go away, elevate your legs and call your doctor right away.

If you have spider veins or if you have larger veins near your skin surface, they definitely are unattractive, but they don't always pose a risk. It's the deep varicose veins in your leg that you might not see that pose a serious problem. If these veins are weak, blood can leak out through their walls and eventually they will burst creating a slow healing ulcer. Or, if a clot is created and breaks loose, it can travel to your lungs, heart or brain causing a serious health issue.

**Varicose Vein Symptoms**

When you have varicose veins you may have a feeling of leg heaviness, cramps at night or a dull aching after standing for a long time. You may also have aching, during your period and feel fatigued. You will have discolored veins visible through your skin. In more severe with deep varicose veins, you can have dark discoloration of the skin or skin ulcers or sores.

With varicose, some people will a have feeling of tightness, congestion, tenderness in the tired legs, and swollen ankles.

**What To Expect From Natural Remedies**

With any natural remedy process, your illness or condition can take a while to improve and this is true when you have varicose veins. You will need to pay constant attention to the natural remedies you use and to the diet and lifestyle changes you need to make that are recommended here. You will need to try the different remedies listed, so you can find out which works for you.

A natural approach to varicose veins will help your varicose veins from getting worse and help you get rid of some of the unwanted appearance.

The reason to use natural remedies for varicose veins is to prevent them from getting worse by changing into phlebitis, where blood clots form on the vein walls.  This is a dangerous life threatening condition which could result in a heart attack or stroke.

When vein valves have been damaged, it is not possible to repair them.  So if your vein valves have been damage, you will not be able to get rid of your varicose veins. But you can prevent them from becoming worse and prevent new ones from forming.  And, you can strengthen the vein walls, so that their appearance is less apparent.

# 2: Do You Know What Causes Varicose Veins?

You have two kinds of blood vessels, arteries and veins. The arteries deliver blood from the heart to all locations in your body. The vein has a more difficult job, because they have to return blood back to your heart.

The arteries move blood through the pumping action of your heart. The veins don't have this help and they have to deliver blood back to your heart, when the muscles surrounding your veins contract and relax.

Exercising can make your muscles contract and force blood back to your heart. Also just ordinary movement of house or office work can help bring blood back into your heart.

**Why is it that you have varicose veins?**

It occurs in both men and women, but more frequently in women. Varicose veins occur when the valves in veins malfunction or when the vein walls weaken. Normally valves only allow the blood to flow in one direction. In this case, the vein valves that exist in the legs are designed to allow blood to flow only upward to the heart.

When you walk, move your legs, or exercise, the muscle around your leg veins contract and force blood upward. When this happens the vein valves open to allow blood to flow upward and then close to prevent that blood from flowing back. When you have varicose veins, the vein valves do not close or do not close enough to prevent the back flow of blood from where it just went. Blood then tends to accumulate in the veins, since it cannot move upward.

When the vein walls are weak, they deform or bulge when blood fills the veins. When the muscles around them contract and expand, the veins cannot hold their structure, because of loss of elasticity. Keeping their form would help to push blood through their valve and back to your heart.

Varicose veins are a result of vein valve malfunction. They are a result of weak valve function and weak vein integrity. Varicose is a symptom of a more serious body condition. One of the main causes of varicose veins is constipation. The severity of your varicose veins is a result of the severity of your constipation and the weakness of your vein walls and valve.

## Constipation

When you have constipation and strain to have a bowel movement, you are putting extra pressure in your abdominal and this in turn puts extra pressure on your leg veins. With this pressure, you are forcing blood back down your legs and passed the vein valves. Forcing blood back down your veins, in the wrong direction, causes the vein valves to become defective. As your constipation continues, this extra pressure, over time, will weaken your veins and vein values, which eventually lead to varicose veins.

## Congested Liver

Varicose veins are related to blood circulation problems. In constipation the blood is forced to flow in the wrong direction damaging the function of the veins and their valves. In the same way, a congested liver can cause varicose veins. All blood moves through the liver. When the liver is congested, it will not pass the amount of blood that is required to circulate throughout your body. The result is that blood backs up putting pressure on your veins and heart valves and this result in varicose veins.

## Deep Varicose Veins

When veins are deep into your leg tissue turn into varicose veins, you may not be aware of this condition, until you begin to see other markings or discoloration on your legs or you feel pain. It's easy to see varicose veins that are near
your skin surface, because they turn a characteristic blue-green color.

Sometimes deep varicose veins display a red, brownish, or white dot on your skin. Skin discoloration should be a warning that you might have serious circulatory problems or heart valves issues that you need to pay attention to.

As your veins swell, your legs and feet can become itchy and sores can develop that become open and appear like ulcer wounds.

**Genetic Vein Wall Weakness**

If you inherit weakness of your vein walls or valves, you will be susceptible to varicose veins. All you need to produce varicose is to be in poor nutritional health. Many people can remember their aunt, mother, or grandmother having varicose. So if you have a history of varicose in your family, then the information here will help you to reduce, prevent, or cure them if they are not too severe.

**Lack Of Minerals**

Minerals are body builders and when you lack them, your body will be weak. In addition, minerals make your body alkaline and when you have an acid body, you create and attract illness and varicose vein are just another illness or condition that comes about from the lack of minerals. Having the right amount of minerals in your body will determine the health of all parts of your body – heart, liver, cardiovascular system, veins, etc.

How do you make sure you have the right amount of minerals in your body? You need to test with litmus paper to see how acidic your body is and then eat those fruits and vegetables that give you an alkaline body.  You can get important information on creating an alkaline body in one of the other books I have written called, "Alkaline Body: Nutrition And Diet Tips."

## Lack of Exercise

The lack of exercise helps to develop varicose veins.  If you sit or stand with little or no movement during the day, you stand a good chance of developing varicose.  You may be sitting at your desk or taking a long flight.  Getting up frequently is a good preventive measure for varicose.

## Long Periods of Standing, Sitting, Or Lifting

If you stand or sit in one position for long periods, blood in your legs will pool.  It tends to collect in your leg veins rather than circulating back to your heart.  It takes leg movements for the blood to flow back up to your heart.  Without this movement, you become more susceptible to varicose veins.

## Damage To Veins or Vein Valves

If you have had any kind of accident that injury's your legs or calves, that injury may weaken your veins.  If this is the case then, this weakness may make you more susceptible to varicose veins.

## Pregnancy

If you are pregnant, the extra weight you have and the hormonal changes you go through will create varicose veins. The extra weight will put pressure on the veins and valves and cause them to stop working properly.

Then blood will flow into small veins that are not designed to carry extra blood. Soon, these veins will stretch forming varicose and become visible through your skin.

## Vein Hardness

Varicose veins just like arteriosclerosis occurs when veins lose their elasticity and become hardened. To recover vein elasticity takes a long time. This can be accomplished by taking vitamin E daily with two tablespoons of lecithin over a period of 3 years. This will soften veins and restore elasticity.

# 3: What Foods Will Fight Your Varicose Veins?

If you want to have nice looking legs without unsightly varicose veins, you need to change your diet into a health one. A diet that will correct or eliminate constipation is what is needed. A diet that will change your acid body into an alkaline body. This type of diet is also great for gaining excellent natural health. A diet for constipation is in the following chapter.

Here are some foods that you should be eating to strengthen your veins. If you have varicose veins, your veins have ballooned out and are weak, so you need to eat those foods and supplements that will strengthen your veins. In addition, you want to improve your blood circulation, so that the nutrients your leg veins need get to your legs.

### Pineapple

Pineapples are great for improving your circulatory and heart condition. It is filled with bromelain, which is an enzyme that helps you digest protein. Eat fresh pineapple 3 times a week. More often if you like it and it is available.

### Buckwheat

Here is a great food to eat for blood circulation. You will need to make sure you get plenty of fiber in your diet and buckwheat has plenty. It contains a flavonoid called rutin, which can strengthen veins. You will find rutin is also available as a supplement.

### Bilberries

Blue-berries or red berries will strengthen the walls of

your veins with the high antioxidant content they have. Use them as snacks between meals, Berries are also good for promoting peristaltic action, which will help you with constipation.

## Garlic and Onions

Use garlic and onions in most of your cooking. They are two of the most powerful herbs that prevent and alleviate disease. They can help you improve your blood and help to prevent blood clotting. Garlic is also effective in restoring the elasticity of hardened veins or arteries.

## Liver Foods

Building up your liver when you have varicose veins is a necessary step. You want to eliminate all possible cause of varicose veins, since you will not know which causes are contributing the most to your condition. So, eat artichokes, dark skinned fruits and berries and their juices – blueberries, cherries, grapes, cherry juice. Take a liver building supplement.

## Cantaloupes

Cantaloupes have an anticlotting factor, which will help you prevent blood clotting in your varicose veins.

## Tomato Juice

Keeping your heart strong and working properly is done by keeping your veins and arteries strong and your blood pure. If you have varicose veins, this puts excess pressure on your heart, so it is in your best interest to reduce or eliminate your varicose condition. Here is a tonic that you can make with tomato juice to feed and strengthen your heart muscles and circulatory system.

1/2 cup of tomato juice

1/2 cup of lemon or orange juice
1 tablespoon of brewer's yeast
6 tablespoons of wheat germ oil

Drink 2 ounces of this mixture 1 hour before your meals.

## Garlic Drink

Juice the following items to create a garlic drink for your varicose veins.

Handful of parsley
1 garlic clove
4 carrots, no green tops
2 stalks of celery

Vary these ingredients to get a juice for your taste.

## Cherry Drink

This cherry drink will help to make you more alkaline, strengthen your veins, and help to keep you normal.

1 cup of pitted cherries
1/4 lime
Bunch of green grapes

# 4: Constipation Remedies That Stop Varicose Veins

To get rid of constipation short term is easy. If you are constipated, you can become regular within a week or two and in some cases a few days. Keeping regular long term is a little harder to do, but you can do it by keeping a healthy diet.

Now here's what you should know and need to do:

Learn how to use your natural body cycles to enhance your body's elimination processes
Drink more water
Add more natural fiber to your diet
Watch that protein, bread, and milk
Eat less processed foods
Eat more fruits and vegetables
Use digestive enzymes and probiotics
Eat good oils
Exercise regularly
Reduce stress and anxiety

**Drink More Water**

This is the first step in getting rid of your constipation. If your stools are hard and you have difficulty getting them out of your rectum, then for sure you need more water or juices. Stools get hard, because:

1. You don't have enough water in your body.

2. They remain too long in your colon and water is sucked out of them and routed back into your blood stream.

3. You have eaten too much fiber from grains, more than 40 gm per day, and not enough fruits and vegetables.

The colon works by pulling water out of your fecal matter as it passes by. It is looking for minerals and other nutrients that can be reuse and it routes them back into your body. If your body doesn't have a lot of water, because you don't drink enough water, it sees fecal matter as a new source of water and pulls it out while it's in the colon.

How much water should you drink? Each person's water requirements are different. However don't force yourself to drink more water. You can start with 4 glasses a day. If you drink that much already then add another glass.

And if you are eating fruits and vegetables as suggested earlier, then you will be getting water from them. If you have pain in the lower left part of your abdomen, because of constipation, drinking water should relieve this pain.

**Add More Fiber To Your Diet**

Start adding more fiber to your diet and as you do, you eventually want to be eating up to 35 grams per day. If you are like most people, you are only getting 8 grams or less of fiber per day.

Eating more whole grains, seeds nuts, vegetables and fruits will give you more fiber. Use grains like wheat, buckwheat and millet. Your diet should be around 70% raw food, until you get control or your eliminate your varicose veins
.
**Here's what fiber in fruits and vegetables do for you:**

One, scraps against your colon walls to keep it clean so that no sticky fecal matter buildup occurs there.

Two, stimulates your colon walls to produce peristaltic movement to move your fecal matter out through your rectum.

Without good peristaltic action you will have constipation.

Three, it keeps moisture in your stools so they don't get too hard and can move easily through the colon.

Four, helps you form bulky stools so they are not runny or extra hard. Stool should not be in short pieces, but should be long.

## Processed Food

All processed foods, such as white flour products, have little or no fiber. Processed foods are found in packages, cans, or bottles. Fiber is removed when various natural flours or grains are processed to make junk food. During this processing, nutrients, vitamins, and minerals are also removed. Only plant foods and lightly processed grains have fiber of varying amounts.

## Morning Body Cycle

Eat fruits, vegetables, fruits juices, vegetables juices, and the most water, between 6 am and noon time. In the morning up to noon, the body is in a elimination and detoxification cycle. You can help it and help yourself by giving it what it needs to complete this detoxification process. It needs liquids, nutrients, and fiber. Fruits and vegetables have up to 70% distilled water.

Fruit and vegetables digest within 45 minutes or less and move quickly into the colon. There they provide liquid, nutrients and fiber that activate peristaltic action.

If you eat protein and carbohydrates in the morning, they take up to 4 hours to digest and this blocks your elimination and detoxification process. This does not allow your colon to cleanse out like it should and you end up with constipation.

## Watch that protein, bread, and milk

Eat less protein, bread, and milk. Protein stays in your stomach up to 4 hours, since it takes a long time to digest. If you don't have enough stomach acid, some of the protein you eat will not get digested. Guess who likes it when you don't digest your protein very good, the bad bacteria in your colon. They thrive on undigested protein and this causes constipation.

Bread in the colon turns to dough and it becomes difficult to move through the colon and out as a stool. Milk has protein that causes mucus throughout your body.

**How to Eat Protein**

If you don't eat vegetables with your protein, this is a big problem. Your protein is going to take a long time going through your colon, or in other words, you will be constipation.

So eat smaller protein portions and always eat it with raw vegetables. The vegetables provide fiber to mix in with the digested protein and you already know why fiber is important in the colon. Don't eat fruit with your meals or as after meal desert. And don't drink anything with your meals, since liquid will dilute your stomach acid.

**How to Eat Bread**

Now, the same is true about bread or other flour products. They digest quicker than protein in the stomach, but in the colon they move very slow. Again, eat them with vegetables unless you want to keep your constipation.

**When's the Best Time to Eat Protein and Carbohydrates**

Now, here is the best way to eat protein and carbohydrates. At lunch or dinner only eat one or the other with raw vegetables.

If you can take it, eat protein and vegetables and no carbohydrates. Or, eat carbohydrates and vegetables and no protein. And, again eat fruits, vegetables, and their juices only in the morning. You can also eat them for afternoon snacks.

Dairy products are associated with constipation. This includes milk, cream soups, cheese, yogurt, and some desserts and baked goods. You can eat some of these foods, but only in small portions.

The best dairy product to eat is cottage cheese. It is the least harmful to the body of all dairy.

## Magnesium

Magnesium, a gentle laxative, helps to prevent constipation by relaxing your colon walls when you are under stress, have anxiety, or have too many worries. It normalizes tension on colon walls allowing normal peristaltic action.

Because magnesium attracts water, you can bring in more water into your colon by taking magnesium supplements or by eating foods, which are high in magnesium. Water in your colon makes your stools softer and allows your colon to absorb water from your fecal matter, if your body needs more water.

How do you know if you are short on magnesium? **You will get** cramps in your calves at night or a so called "Charlie horse." Or, you will feel sore after some mild exercise or activity.

Take 400 mg in the morning and 400 mg in the evening of Magnesium gluconate, or citrate. And, of course, take it with calcium. Take the same amount of calcium as you do magnesium. Start with 200 mg at bedtime or you may want to start with 600 – 800 mg.

## Fish Oil

Fish oil contains omega-3 fatty acids, which are essential for good health. It has these fatty acids in the form of EPA, eicosapentaenoic acid and DHA, docosahexaenoic acid.

Fatty acids help reduce inflammation through prostaglandin production. Prostaglandin's help reduces inflammation in your colon, which helps make your colon work better and reduces the possibility of constipation.

Use the enteric-coated fish oil capsules to reduce colon inflammation and to help reduce constipation.

Make sure when taking fish oil that is it is not fish liver oil. They are not the same food product. Fish oil can elevate blood sugar and cholesterol levels in some diabetics.

**Eat More Fruits and Vegetables**

Fruits are made by nature and are a perfect food. They contain the right balance of nutrients with about 70% or more of distilled water. You gain enormous benefits from eating fruits, especially if you eat the outer skin. Eat them without cooking them. They are easy to digest and absorb and do not stress your colon. They activate peristaltic action in the colon and help you have a bowel movement. If you eat them during breaks you will have less constipation.

 **Here are some of the fruits to eat:**

Apples
Apricots
Avocados
Bananas
Blueberries
Boysenberries
Cantaloupes
Cherries
Figs and dates
Grapes

Grapes
Lemons
Nectarines
Oranges
Papayas
Peaches
Pears
Persimmons
Plums
Prunes
Raspberries
Strawberries
Watermelons

**Salt**

Use the least salt as you can in your food. You need salt in your diet, but not as much as people normally add to their food. Salt attracts water, inside your body. Excess salt can create edema in your legs and this would increase the pressure in your leg veins and this is not what you want, if you want to reduce or eliminate varicose veins.

# 5: How Varicose Veins Are Created By An Acid Body

### Minerals

Moving your body more toward alkalinity is what will help you lose weight. If you have an acid body, it will be hard to lose weight. An acid body attracts disease, pathogens, and water, which produces toxins that can be stored as fat. In addition, a diseased body is associated with being overweight and lacking the proper nutrition.

An alkaline body prevents your body from becoming ill and forming deadly diseases, like all kinds of joint problems, organ degradation, body pain, heart disease, or even cancer. If you are already sick, then all of the chemicals inside fruits will help to revive you to better health. This is provided that your tissue damage has not gone beyond repair.

The minerals most important in changing and maintaining your body in an alkaline condition are sodium, potassium, chloride, calcium, phosphorus, magnesium, and sulphur.

Now, how your body can become alkaline might become a little confusing at first because of the terms used, but let's break this down into small parts. First we are going to be defining some terms, so we can then start talking the same language

### Acid Binding

There are certain minerals that are called acid binding. And these are minerals we said are the most important ones in fruits - Sodium, potassium, chloride, calcium, phosphorus, and magnesium - because they are acid binding.

What acid binding means is when you eat fruits with these minerals, they will combine with acids in your body and neutralize them. These neutralized acids will be then be eliminated from your body in your urine and feces.

If not all the acid toxins are captured by acid binding matter, the remaining acids can be neutralized by body stores of alkaline minerals. If you don't have a good store of alkaline minerals, then these acids will remain in your body creating disease. But if you do have a good store of alkaline minerals, these minerals will find acids, capture them, and bind with them. Then these acids will be moved out of your body, by your urine, stools, and breath.

So you can see the importance of getting a lot of alkaline minerals into your body. Without them, acids would not get eliminate from your body, and they would remain in your body tissue and continue their body damage.

Acid binding minerals mainly come from eating vegetables and fruits.

**Alkaline Binding**

Now, there are also minerals that become alkaline binding and these minerals are sulphur, chlorine, iodine, phosphorus, bromine, fluorine, copper, and silicon. It is these minerals that when digested by a cell will produce a salt that will bind with alkaline minerals. These minerals will be excreted through your urine.

When alkaline minerals are trapped by an acid salt, the alkaline mineral is removed from your body and your body becomes more acidic. This is the condition you are trying to avoid.

Foods that are alkaline binding and remove the minerals that you need to make your body alkaline are meat, carbohydrates, some vegetables and some fruits.

Although you need to eat both foods that are acid binding or alkaline binding, you want to eat more of the acid binding foods. This will keep your body slightly alkaline.

## Where do Acid Toxins Come From?

So why is the body overloaded with toxins? Why can't the liver take care of these toxins? Your liver has the function to remove acid wastes from natural food that is created by food digestion and cell metabolism. When your body encounters acid wastes, such as food enhancers, dyes, preservatives, pesticides, and the variety of additives, the liver does not know how to break them down or make them harmless.

But your body does not give up so easily, when it knows that the liver is not able to disintegrate food additives. What it does is it instructs calcium to bind with these toxic
acids and to take them far away from the blood stream.

Now, we have talked about acid toxins in the body that are brought in through food and the environment. But there is another factor that creates acid in the body and that is emotions that are activated through life stresses, like work pressures, divorce, friendship problems, martial issues, and other similar situations. These emotional problems create acidic molecules that then embed themselves into your tissues just like food acids. These again can be removed with minerals.

## Body Organs

All body organs function to rid the body of acid waste or toxins. Lack of acid binding food causes the deterioration of these organs. Each organ has a specific function in the elimination and neutralization of acid wastes and it does this in conjunction with acid binding minerals.

## Acid Binding Foods

Here is a list of the fruits that have the highest alkaline minerals and the ones that you should be eating to eliminate your body acids.

The percentage assigned to these fruits is based on fresh fruits that are organic and that they are not cooked, canned or mixed with sugar. If they are cook or otherwise processed in some fashion, this will reduce their effectiveness as an acid binding fruit. However, they will still be somewhat effective in acid binding.

Fruits above 50% in value are more acid binding, which means they will trap acid wastes better. You will want to eat and drink those fruits above 51%.

The fruits that are at 50% at are neutral. They are not acid binding nor alkaline binding.

Here is the list of fruits to eat and drink in the order of priority.

1. Fruits at 100% Acid Binding – Best fruits To Eat And Drink
Lemons, melons – any type, watermelon

2. Fruits at 93% Acid Binding – Great fruits To Eat and Drink
Cantaloupes, dried dates, dried figs, limes, mango, papaya

3. Fruits at 87% Acid Binding – Still Great Fruits to Eat and Drink
Kiwis, passion fruit, pineapples, raisins, umeboshi plums

4. Fruits at 80% Acid Binding – Eat And Drink These Fruits
Apricots, avocados, bananas, fresh dates, fresh figs, currants, gooseberries grapes, grapefruits guavas, kumquats, nectarines, pears, persimmons, quince

5.     Fruits at 73% Acid Binding – Still Fruits To Eat And Drink
Apples, organs, peaches, pomegranate, raspberries, sour grapes, strawberries

6.     Fruits at 67% Acid Binding – Still Neutralizes Acids, Eat And Drink This fruit
Cherries

**Fruits to Concentrate On**

These are the fruits you should concentrate on eating. Also eat them every day, if possible, fresh lemon juice in the morning, watermelon during the day.

You can see which fruits give you the best acid binding effects and eating and drinking them 80% of your overall food intake will convert your body over to an Alkaline body.

# 6: Most Powerful Supplements for Varicose Veins

Here some of the better and most powerful supplements that you can use to help you with your varicose veins. These supplements will improve your blood circulation, strengthen your vein walls, and improve your overall cardiovascular system.

**Glycosaminoglycans (GAGs)**

Here is a group of nutrients that has been found to be more effective in treating varicose vein than most other nutrients. You can get these nutrients through the Enzymatic Therapy Brand. The product is call Better Veins, but was called Aorta-Glycan. You can go to the internet to check out this product. Use this product in combination with many other supplement and herbs listed to create a powerful approach to getting relief from your varicose veins.

**Bromelain**

Here is an enzyme that can breakdown the fibrin that accumulates around varicose veins. Get bromelain at a health food store and take 500mg twice a day, before meals or in between meals.

**Quercetin-C**

Quercetin-C is a bioflavonoid and can be found at your health food store. It has been shown to prevent and relieve varicose veins. It helps to reduce the feeling of fatigue and heaviness in your legs. In addition, it reduces the permeability of capillaries, which reduces the amount of fluids that pass through your capillary walls. Take 1000 mg daily.

## Cayenne Pepper

Cayenne pepper is an amazing herb and provides nutrients that can strengthen your heart, veins, and balance your circulation system. Follow the instructions on the bottle. Typically you should take capsules 2 to 3 times a day and they should be taken with meals. You will feel a slight hotness in your stomach, when you first start to take them. If you like hot foods all chilies help to improve your cardiovascular system.

## Chlorophyll

Chlorophyll is similar to the hemoglobin molecule in your blood, except that at the center of the hemoglobin molecule is the mineral iron and the chlorophyll center is magnesium. So, if you want to build your blood, drinking chlorophyll is one way to do it.

Drinking chlorophyll will help increase the hemoglobin in your blood. By drinking chlorophyll you will rejuvenate your blood and revitalize your veins in your legs. You can buy liquid chlorophyll at your health food store. Drink it first thing in the morning. Place a tablespoon or two in a glass of water and squeeze 1/2 lemon juice into the glass. Then drink up and if the taste is not to your liking, add the chlorophyll to a fruit juice.

## Footbaths

Footbaths have been found to help reduce that appearance, pain and sluggishness of varicose veins. The footbath is easy to use and relaxing. Do it 20 minutes a day after your work day. Here how to do it.

Heat a quart of water to boiling, the turn off the heat. Place some of the herbs listed here and let them sit for 30 minutes – garlic, horse chestnut, oatstraw, bayberry, butcher's broom, hyssop, etc. Just try different combinations, they will not hurt you. Turn on your footbath and bring the water to hot and add your drained and filtered herbal mixture. You're ready to turn on the bubble and put your feet into your footbath.

## Vitamin E

Vitamin E is good for preventing blood clots, reducing circulatory problems, and rebuilding the vein walls. You can get vitamin in wheat germ or in capsule form. Use 800 to 1,200 IU, 500 in the morning and 500 in the evening. If you start to feel uncomfortable sensation, when starting on vitamin E, there is no need to worry. This is typical when using it for varicose veins.

## Flaxseed oil

This oil will help you with constipation by reducing the strain and force you use for a bowel movement. You can use 1 to 2 tablespoons per day. You can use it in your salads, cereals, smoothies, and soups when ready to eat.

## Lecithin

You can get lecithin in granules. Use 2 teaspoons or more every day. It has very little taste and can be added to your salads, cereal, or soups. Lecithin helps to break up fat in your blood and to reduce the amount of plaque that builds up along your arteries. This is an easy supplement to use and you should incorporate it into your diet.

## Milk Thistle

Milk thistle is the major herb that has nutrients to support liver function. You need to have a strong liver to prevent varicose veins due to a congested liver. The other herbs that support the liver are dandelion root, bilberry extract, red clover and Gotu kola. Get a good liver complex like, Liver Support, **Quantum.** This product has the best herbs for liver support and health.

## MSM

MSM capsules will helps to reduce inflammation cause by varicose veins. When you have inflammation in a specific area, it is hard for that area to heal. Healing starts to take place when inflammation is reduce or eliminated. When inflammation lessens in varicose veins, you will be able to stand longer.

## Oatstraw Tea

Oatstraw tea is excellent to strengthen veins and to help reduce their rigidity. Use 1 ounce of oat straw herb in 1 quart boiling water. Let it sit for 1/2 hour and then drink this in place of water.

## Vitamin C

Vitamin C is used to strengthen your veins and capillaries. Use 3000 to 4000 mg daily but break it up into 3 doses. This is an important vitamin to take, since you need it to have strong vein walls.

## Zinc

Zinc aids in healing of varicose veins. You can take around 20 mg per day.

# 7: Effective Natural Remedies For Varicose Veins

**Apple Cider Vinegar**

Using apple cider vinegar can help you shrink your varicose veins. With a cotton swab rub on 100% apple cider vinegar the whole length of your varicose vein, morning and night.

Also every day drink 2 to 3 glasses of water with two teaspoons of apple cider vinegar. This cider is high in the minerals that help make your body alkaline and to strengthen your viens.

Avoid using regular vinegar; it contains 3 to 9% acetic acid. This acid has been found to contribute to the hardening of the liver and to cause intestinal ulcers.

**Bayberry**

Bayberry is good for blood circulation. You can use it to soothe inflamed varicose veins. You can use it in capsule form. For your skin in the varicose area, use an extract or powder. Mix 10 to 20 drops in water and with a cotton ball apply it to your skin. In powder form, mix ½ teaspoon in ½ cup warm water.

You can use it as a formentation. Place a moisture absorbent towel or cloth into bayberry tea. Place onto your skin as hot as you can tolerate it. Place another cloth over the wet herb cloth and place a heating pad or hot water bottle on top of this cloth. Keep it there for 20 minutes or so. The tea can be made with one tablespoon of bayberry bark placed into boiling water. Then take tea off the hot plate and let sit for 30 minutes before you use it.

**Bilberries**

Bilberries reduce the production of lysosomal enzymes, which contribute to varicose veins. Blue-berries are filled with antioxidants, which make your vein walls strong. This herb like many other herbs improves blood circulation through veins. Recommended dose for bilberry is 240 mg to 480 mg divided in three parts during the day.

## Butcher's Broom

This Mediterranean herb has long been used for varicose veins. In an Italian study, people with varicose veins, which had leg pain, swelling, and itching got improvement after 2 months with butcher's broom. Even though the dose was low at 16.5 mg with vitamin C, these people still saw results. These supplements are now available in 500 mg. Take the dose recommended on the product bottle.

Butcher's broom side effects can be upset stomach and diarrhea. Do not use this herb when taking blood thinning drugs. If you are taking drugs, check with your doctor before using butcher's broom.

## Calendula Salve

Here is a salve that was made by an herbalist that claims to have cleared or cure varicose veins. Yes, there are some cases where specific natural remedies have made varicose veins disappear, but their disappearance has to do with the individual's health, the severity of the varicose veins, the natural remedy used, how often the remedy was used, and the state of mind of the individual being treated.

Here is the salve that was made:

Chop two large handfuls of fresh calendula leaves, flowers and stems. Melt 2.5 cups of lard and add the calendula. Stir together for a few minutes. Remove the pan from the heat and let sit for 24 hours. The next day warm the mixture and filter contents through a cloth. Store the mixture in small jars. Use this salve in the areas of your varicose veins. Lard is very absorbent through your skin and it will deliver the nutrients of calendula into the areas of your varicose veins.

## Fibrin Remedies

When you have varicose veins, fibrin will deposit around these veins giving you lumpy skin. In addition it makes the areas around the vein hard and this contributes to pain. Fibrin forms throughout your body and is detrimental in excess, but in the vein area it is trying to reduce inflammation of the veins.

When fibrin gets out of control, it will over deposits on the veins preventing them from functioning properly and from getting back to normal. To eliminate this fibrin use garlic, onions and ground red pepper in your cooking. Another way to get these foods into your body is to use a footbath.

You can also use a product called Neprinol. This product consists of what is called "systemic enzymes." These enzymes are coated so they reach the small intestine, where they are digested and enter your blood. These enzymes are designed to get into your blood and breakdown fibrin wherever it finds.

Neprinol contains serrapeptase, nattokinase, lipase, papain, bromelain rutin, protease, amia, magnesium, and Co-Q10.

Another systemic enzyme system you can use is called Vitalzyn, which is also good.

## Ginkgo Biloba

Ginkgo helps to increase blood flow to peripheral arteries and heart. It also helps protect blood vessels, prevents leaking from small veins, and prevents some blood clotting. Take 40mg three times a day of extract standardized to 24% ginkgo flavone glycosides and 6% terpene lactones.

## Gotu Kola

In a condition called venous insufficiency, which is more serious than varicose veins, Gotu cola was found by European studies to improve this condition. Venous insufficiency occurs in deep veins in the legs and elsewhere in your body. Gotu cola helps to strengthen your veins and vein valves, so they work better in both venous insufficiency and varicose veins. In this study, 60 and 120 mg were used.

Both doses worked better than the placebo, but the 120 mg work best of all. The recommended dose for this herb is quite a bit higher. Take 2,000 to 3,000 mg three times a day in capsule form for varicose veins. Gauge how much to use based on what improvement you see in your varicose veins. If you see some improvement, use a little more until you get the improvement you want.

**Grape Seed Extra, Pine Bark Extract**

Grape seed extra has a nutrient called procyanidolic oligomers, which has been found to be effective in treating varicose veins. It is widely used in Europe for this condition.

**Ginger**

Ginger also helps to break down fibrin that surrounds the varicose veins. If you have varicose veins, you will have lost a lot of your ability to break down fibrin. So take those nutrients and products listed for eliminating fibrin.

**Hawthorn**

This herb can be use to strengthen and protect your whole cardiovascular system. It is high in antioxidant, so it helps to lower your blood pressure and prevents clotting. Varicose veins can sometimes creating blood clots in its advanced states.

**Horse Chestnut Seeds (Buckeye)**

Horse chestnut (aesculus hippocastanum) has long been used for treating varicose veins. These seeds contain a compound call escin, which strengthens your veins and make them more elastic, by sealing off tiny openings in your vein walls. This helps your veins to have healthier blood flow. This herb can also relieve the itching and pain associated with your varicose.

Use around 300 mg every 12 hours for up to 12 weeks. Use a standardized extract of horse chestnut herb that contains up to 75 mg of escin per dose.

A cream or gel is also available for horse chestnut, which contain 2% escin. You apply it to your skin 3-4 times daily. Wash your hands before and after applying this cream. Gently apply a thin layer to the varicose area. Do not get it into your eyes, nose or broken skin. Keep away from children, since it can be toxic.

If you are using any blood thinners, do not use horse chestnut, since it also thins your blood. If you are diabetic, it could lower you blood sugar, so check your sugar regularly, if you decide to use this herb.

If you can't find a cream in the USA, you can make your own. Mix ½ teaspoon of horse chestnut powder into 16 ounces of water. Softly apply this solution into the varicose area. If you have MSM add 2000 mg powder or hard capsules to this solution and wait for it to dissolve, before you use it.

**Hyssop Formulation**

Here is an herb formulation to take for varicose veins. Collect 1 ounce of the following herbs. If you have a capsule maker, you can buy the powdered herbs and make your own capsules.

Powdered hyssop
Yellow dock root
Bayberry bark
Boneset

Wood sage

In a quart of water boil this herb mixture for 1/2 hours. Strain and drink a glass right before meals.

## Persimmon juice

Take the juice of persimmon and place it on a cotton ball. Then rub this juice onto your legs where varicose exist. Do this every day. This should prevent your varicose from becoming worse.

## Rutin

Rutin is a flavonoid that is found in many foods and can strengthen your vein walls. You can find rutin in capsules or you can find it mixed with other flavonoids in capsules. You can take 500 mg of rutin daily.

## Anthocyanidins

Anthocyanidins are nutrients found in blueberries, purple grapes, or other fruits with deep color. It is these nutrients that give the fruit its color. Anthocyanidins protect vein walls and prevent blood or plasma from leaking out of the walls. They also strengthen the connective tissue that supports the blood vessels. You can take 150 mg per day.

## Witch Hazel

Witch hazel is an anti-inflammatory solution which you can use several times a day. Use witch hazel as an extract, gel or cream. Rub it in the affect leg area, but do not rub hard. To massage, only massage around the affected area not directly. You can make a wet compress using witch hazel and apply it to the area needed. For an effective witch hazel product look for a Nondistilled Hydroalcoholic Extract. This may be hard to find.

## Yarrow Tea

Use yarrow tea morning and night. Yarrow will cleanse your blood and liver and this will help you recover or prevent varicose veins. You can also use yarrow as a poultice on severe cases of varicose.

## Cellu-Var

Here is an herbal formulation that contains butchers broom, rhizome extract, horse chestnut extract, and Gotu kola. It's a convenient herbal mixture to help you treat your varicose veins.

# 8: Final Comments On Varicose Veins

There you have it. There are a lot of different remedies that you can use. Look them over and start using the ones that fit the symptoms you want to get rid of. Choose 3 or 4 of them and start using them. Use them for a month to see what results you get.

If you get good results then keep using them for 3 months, then replace one remedy with another one at the end of 3 month. If you see no results choose another 3 to work with. Keep working with the different remedies.

Also use some of the external salves or creams and at the same time use the internal remedies.

Make sure you follow the different constipation and alkaline diets that are provided. It is critical that you move your body from acid to alkaline. Here are some other things to use and follow.

### Calcium and Magnesium

Use calcium citrate 500mg and magnesium citrate 1500mg to relieve the night pain and discomfort of your varicose veins. Take this combination just before you go to bed so you can improve your sleep.

Here are some sensible things to do to improve your blood circulation in your legs. Remember that when blood in your legs is not allowed to move up your body, you become susceptible to varicose.

### Weight Loss

If you are overweight, this will put more weight and pressure on your legs.  This pressure will prevent a lot of blood in your legs from circulating properly.  You will need to lose weight.  This may be difficult to do, since there are so many weight loss programs that people use that do not work or work for a while and then the weight comes back.  Look at what is required to get an alkaline body.  Follow this information and you will lose weight.  In addition, I have created a new weight loss program called, "Ten (10) Day Quick Success Weight Loss Program."  This is a new way of losing weight and keeping it off.

## Clothing

Don't wear clothes that are too tight around your waist, since this will obstruct your circulation.  When you have pressure about your stomach area, it is harder for blood to return from your legs to your heart.

## Stockings and Heels

You can wear support hose to give you some relief from varicose veins, but don't depend on this to be a cure.  You can buy the best hose in a pharmacy or medical supply house.  Make use of some of the remedies and techniques mentioned here to reduce your varicose.  Also try not to use high-heel shoes until you get your varicose veins under control.  Heels put a lot of muscle stress on your calves.  Or, just try to use heels less frequent.

## Standing

If you have to stand a long time, rock back and forth on your legs.  This allows some leg muscle contractions to circulate your blood upward.

## Your Bed

You can raise your bed by 6 inches, so that your legs will be elevated. This will help your blood to flow away from your legs, giving you relief from aching legs.

**Elevating Your Legs**

To get better blood flow from your legs to your heart, raise your legs above your heart in a sitting position. This helps to circulate blood from your legs to your heart and heal your varicose veins. It removes the some of pressure off of your circulatory system. Swelling in your legs will go down and healing will start.

**Exercise**

Sitting all day can be a factor in how varicose veins are formed. If you sit or stand in one place during the day, your leg muscles don't contract much. If you sit, get up every once in a while and walk around or exercise your legs. The same is true if you stand in one place. If you can move around a little bit so your leg muscles are not under constant pressure.

Or, try to keep your feet active during the day. You can raise yourself up and down on your toes. Do a few deep knee bends when possible. Shake your legs on occasion. Rotate your feet. Do anything that helps to keep your legs active and not standing or sitting all day.

If you have time, do some walking before work or after. Walking or doing leg exercises get your blood moving in your legs and helps to strengthen both your leg muscles and leg veins. Walking, riding a bike, jogging, rebounding, or any exercise or activity that contracts your leg muscles will help to push pooled blood in your legs back into circulation.

The best exercise for varicose veins is bicycling or a stationary exercise bike. Swimming is another great exercise. If you can do this several time a week that would be good.

Another exercise to do is to lie in bed and raise your legs and move them as if riding a bicycle for 5 minutes and twice a day if possible. If you can do a head stand for 3 minutes morning and night, this is also helpful. A yoga position where you lie on your back and raise your legs with your torso up in the air is also good.

Any exercise where you feel a stretch in your ankles and calves is a good exercise for varicose veins.

# 9: Resources You Need To Know About

Thank you for taking time to read my e-book. I sincerely hope that there are some remedies and procedures here that will help give you relief and hopefully a cure for your varicose veins. Here are some additional e-books that I have written that will also help you gain better health.

Rudy Silva is a natural consultant nutritionist educated in the United State in Nutrition and Physics. He is a graduate from the University Of San Jose State in California. He is author of 20 other e-books on natural remedies. He has authored a newsletter in natural remedies for over 4 years. He has many websites promoting special recommended products and information.

He is now living in the Philippines where he writes nutrition and remedy e-books.

## Resource page

Here is other kindle e-book about using natural remedies that have been written by this author.

## http://tinyurl.com/b2f7wd3

### Acne Remedies
Best natural acne treatments: Acne facial

### Constipation Remedies
Best Constipated Women Natural Cures
How To Relieve Constipation With Fruits

### Essential Fatty Acids
Taking The Mystery Out Of Essential Fatty acids

Amazing Fish Oil Benefits Revealed

## Nutrition Remedies
Updated Version - Secret Diet And Nutrition
Secret Healthy Fruit Practices Revealed
Fast Healing Juice Nutrition Therapy: Nutrition Tips 3
Fantastic Alkaline Fruit Benefits Revealed
Calcium (Discover How To Use Calcium To Avoid Devastating Diseases)
Magnesium Nutrition Revealed
Best Nutrition Health Practices
Potassium Health Secrets Revealed
Phosphorus, The Best Brain Food
**A Sodium Diet (What You Must Know About Sodium)**
**Vegetables and Vegetable Juice Cures**

## Stomach Remedies
Acid Reflux: Fast and Easy Cures For Acid Reflux
Asthma Treatment Cures With Remedies
How To Do Natural Colon Cleansing
Gastrointestinal Digestion Secrets Revealed

## Misc Remedies
Natural Hair Loss Treatment: Women And Men
Effective Natural Hemorrhoids Treatment
Iron Deficiency Anemia
Secrets To Understanding Behavior
Fast Acting Ear Infection Remedies
Best Impotence Health Diet
What Is A Hiatus Hernia
Best Varicose Vein Treatments?

## Men's Health
Best Impotence Health Diet

## Weight loss
Ten (10) Day Quick Success Weight Loss Program: A new approach to losing weight by changing your eating habits for life

To see all of the kindle books written by this author, go to this the Authors Profile Page or this URL: http://tinyurl.com/b2f7wd3

If you need support or want to promote any of his e-books, please contact him at rss41@yahoo.com and expect a reply within 24 hours. He looks forward to hearing from you and is happy to help you understand his material on natural and nutritional health.

**Give A Review**

And, don't for get to give a review for this e-book at Amazon so that others can gain the benefits of what is in this e-book.

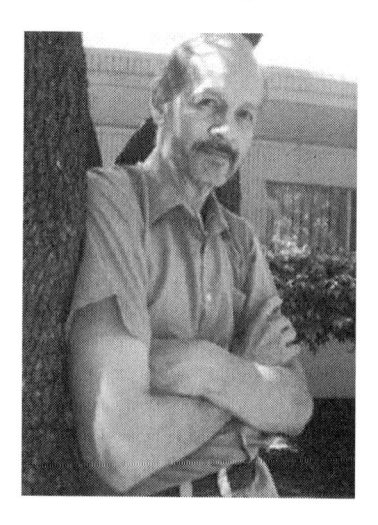

To you, for creating better health and more happiness in your life,

*Rudy S Silva*

Rudy S Silva, Natural Nutritionist

Printed in Great Britain
by Amazon